A Beginner's Guide to Neutrino Physics: From Basics to Advanced Concepts

Alexia

Copyright © [2023]

Title: A Beginner's Guide to Neutrino Physics: From Basics to Advanced Concepts

Author's: Alexia.

All rights reserved. No part of this publication may be reproduced, stored in a retrieval system, or transmitted in any form or by any means, electronic, mechanical, photocopying, recording, or otherwise, without the prior written permission of the publisher or author, except in the case of brief quotations embodied in critical reviews and certain other non-commercial uses permitted by copyright law.

This book was printed and published by [Publisher's: Alexia] in [2023]

ISBN:

TABLE OF CONTENTS

Chapter 1: Introduction to Neutrino Physics
06

The Discovery of Neutrinos

Properties of Neutrinos

Neutrino Interactions

Chapter 2: Neutrino Oscillations 13

Neutrino Flavor States

The Pontecorvo-Maki-Nakagawa-Sakata (PMNS) Matrix

Neutrino Oscillation Experiments

Chapter 3: Neutrino Sources and Detection
19

Neutrino Sources: Solar, Atmospheric, and Supernovae

Neutrino Detection Techniques: Scintillation Detectors and Cherenkov Radiation

Neutrino Observatories: IceCube, Super-Kamiokande, and Others

Chapter 4: Neutrino Mass and Mixing   25

Neutrino Mass Hierarchy

Absolute Neutrino Mass Measurements

Leptogenesis and Neutrino Mass

Chapter 5: Neutrino Interactions with Matter   31

Charged Current and Neutral Current Interactions

Neutrino-Nucleus Scattering

Neutrino-Electron Scattering

Chapter 6: Neutrino Phenomenology   37

Neutrino Physics Beyond the Standard Model

Neutrinoless Double Beta Decay

Neutrino Astrophysics: Supernovae and Neutrino Astronomy

Chapter 7: Neutrino Experiments and Future Prospects   44

Current Neutrino Experiments: Daya Bay, T2K, and NOvA

Future Neutrino Experiments: DUNE, Hyper-Kamiokande, and JUNO

Neutrino Physics at Colliders: The Long-Baseline Neutrino Facility (LBNF)

Chapter 8: Applications of Neutrino Physics 50

Neutrinos and Particle Astrophysics

Neutrinos in Cosmology

Neutrinos and Dark Matter

Chapter 9: Open Questions and Challenges in Neutrino Physics 56

Neutrino Mass Ordering

CP Violation in Neutrino Oscillations

Neutrino Physics and the Nature of Dark Matter

Chapter 10: Conclusion 63

Summary of Key Concepts

The Future of Neutrino Physics

Chapter 1: Introduction to Neutrino Physics

The Discovery of Neutrinos

In the vast realm of particle physics, one of the most intriguing and elusive particles is the neutrino. The discovery of neutrinos revolutionized our understanding of the fundamental building blocks of the universe. In this subchapter, we delve into the captivating story behind the detection and characterization of these mysterious particles.

The journey to unravel the secrets of neutrinos began in the early 20th century. In 1930, physicist Wolfgang Pauli proposed the existence of a neutral particle that could explain the missing energy and momentum in certain radioactive decays. Pauli named this hypothetical particle the "neutrino," which means "little neutral one" in Italian.

Years later, in 1956, the first experimental evidence for neutrinos emerged. A team of scientists led by Clyde Cowan and Frederick Reines conducted the famous neutrino detection experiment at the Savannah River nuclear reactor in South Carolina. This innovative experiment involved observing the interaction between neutrinos and protons, resulting in the detection of electron antineutrinos. Cowan and Reines' groundbreaking work confirmed the existence of neutrinos and earned them the Nobel Prize in Physics in 1995.

Since then, numerous experiments have expanded our knowledge of neutrinos. These elusive particles come in three flavors: electron, muon, and tau neutrinos. They possess minuscule masses, making them difficult to detect and study. However, their intriguing properties have captivated scientists worldwide.

Neutrinos have played a crucial role in unraveling the mysteries of the universe. They are produced in various astrophysical phenomena, such as supernovae and black holes, and carry valuable information about these cosmic events. Moreover, neutrinos have been instrumental in understanding the phenomenon of neutrino oscillation, whereby they change from one flavor to another as they travel through space.

The study of neutrinos has also led to profound implications beyond particle physics. Neutrino experiments have shed light on the nature of matter and antimatter asymmetry in the universe. Furthermore, they have provided insights into the fundamental properties of neutrinos, such as their masses and mixing angles.

As we delve deeper into the intricacies of neutrino physics, we unlock new frontiers and pave the way for groundbreaking discoveries. From neutrino telescopes buried deep underground to detectors submerged in vast bodies of water, scientists continue to push the boundaries of our knowledge. The study of neutrinos promises to unravel the secrets of the universe and revolutionize our understanding of particle physics.

In this subchapter, we have embarked on a journey through time, exploring the captivating story behind the discovery of neutrinos. From Pauli's theoretical proposal to the pioneering experiments of Cowan and Reines, we have witnessed the birth of a new field of physics. The enigma of neutrinos continues to inspire scientists and captivate the imagination of enthusiasts worldwide, reminding us of the limitless wonders that lie within the realm of particle physics.

Properties of Neutrinos

Neutrinos are fundamental particles that play a crucial role in our understanding of the universe. In this subchapter, we will explore the properties of neutrinos, shedding light on their mysterious nature and their significance in the field of particle physics.

First and foremost, neutrinos are electrically neutral, meaning they carry no electric charge. This property allows them to interact only through the weak nuclear force, making them extremely elusive and difficult to detect. In fact, neutrinos can pass through matter without any interaction, making them essentially invisible. This unique characteristic has led scientists to refer to neutrinos as "ghost particles."

The second property of neutrinos that sets them apart from other particles is their extremely low mass. While the exact mass of neutrinos is still uncertain, it is known to be much lighter than any other known particle. This property has significant implications for cosmology and the formation of the universe. Additionally, the small mass of neutrinos causes them to travel at nearly the speed of light, allowing them to traverse vast distances in a short amount of time.

Neutrinos come in three different types, or flavors, known as electron neutrinos, muon neutrinos, and tau neutrinos. Each flavor is associated with a corresponding charged lepton (electron, muon, or tau). However, neutrinos have the intriguing ability to oscillate between different flavors as they travel through space. This phenomenon, known as neutrino oscillation, was discovered through groundbreaking experiments and has revolutionized our understanding of particle physics.

Another fascinating property of neutrinos is their involvement in some of the most energetic and violent events in the universe. Neutrinos are produced in abundance during supernovae, gamma-ray bursts, and other cosmic phenomena. By studying these neutrinos, scientists can gain valuable insights into the inner workings of such cataclysmic events.

Understanding the properties of neutrinos is not only important for the field of particle physics but also has implications for cosmology, astrophysics, and even the search for dark matter. Neutrinos provide a window into the hidden aspects of the universe, offering a unique perspective on the fundamental forces and particles that shape our world.

In conclusion, neutrinos possess a variety of unique properties that make them one of the most intriguing particles in the universe. Their electric neutrality, low mass, flavor oscillation, and involvement in cosmic events make them a fascinating subject of study for scientists across various disciplines. By unraveling the mysteries of neutrinos, we can unlock a deeper understanding of the fundamental workings of our universe.

Neutrino Interactions

In the exciting field of particle physics, the study of neutrinos has attracted much attention in recent years. These tiny, elusive particles have a fascinating nature and play a significant role in shaping our understanding of the fundamental building blocks of the universe. In this subchapter, we will delve into the intriguing world of neutrino interactions, shedding light on their behavior and the implications they have for the field of particle physics.

Neutrinos, often referred to as "ghost particles," are incredibly lightweight and chargeless, making them notoriously difficult to detect. However, their unique properties allow them to interact weakly with other particles, providing scientists with a means to study them indirectly. Neutrino interactions occur through the weak nuclear force, one of the four fundamental forces of nature, alongside gravity, electromagnetism, and the strong nuclear force.

The weak nuclear force governs processes such as radioactive decay and plays a vital role in the fusion reactions occurring within the sun. Neutrinos, being weakly interacting, readily participate in weak interactions, making them ideal probes to study various phenomena in particle physics. By observing these interactions, scientists can unravel mysteries such as the nature of neutrino masses, their oscillation behavior, and the possibility of new physics beyond the Standard Model.

Neutrino interactions come in different flavors: electron neutrinos, muon neutrinos, and tau neutrinos. As neutrinos propagate through space, they can oscillate between these flavors, a phenomenon known as neutrino oscillation. This oscillation provides insights into the properties and masses of neutrinos, offering a window into the inner workings of the universe.

Understanding neutrino interactions is crucial for experiments designed to study these elusive particles. Experiments like the Super-Kamiokande, IceCube, and DUNE aim to detect neutrinos and study their properties. By observing the interactions of neutrinos with various target materials, scientists can decipher crucial information about their energy, momentum, and scattering angles.

Neutrino interactions not only contribute to our understanding of fundamental particles but also have implications for astrophysics and cosmology. Neutrinos produced in the core of the sun, in cosmic ray interactions, or during supernova explosions carry valuable information about these astrophysical phenomena. Studying these interactions can unlock secrets about the universe's evolution, the formation of galaxies, and the existence of dark matter and dark energy.

In conclusion, neutrino interactions are a fascinating area of study within particle physics. These weakly interacting particles provide invaluable insights into the fundamental nature of our universe. By observing their interactions, scientists can unravel mysteries ranging from neutrino oscillations to the composition and evolution of the cosmos. Neutrino physics continues to be an exciting field with the potential to revolutionize our understanding of the universe and the fundamental particles that make it up.

Chapter 2: Neutrino Oscillations

Neutrino Flavor States

In the fascinating realm of particle physics, one particular enigmatic particle has captured the imagination of scientists and enthusiasts alike: the neutrino. These elusive particles, often referred to as "ghost particles," have intrigued researchers for decades due to their peculiar properties and their potential to unlock the mysteries of the universe. In this subchapter, we delve into the concept of neutrino flavor states, shedding light on this fundamental aspect of neutrino physics.

Neutrinos come in three different flavors: electron neutrinos, muon neutrinos, and tau neutrinos. Each flavor corresponds to a different charged lepton - the electron, the muon, and the tau. However, the behavior of neutrinos is far from straightforward. Unlike their charged lepton counterparts, neutrinos can oscillate or change their flavor as they propagate through space.

This phenomenon of neutrino oscillation is a result of the quantum mechanical nature of these subatomic particles. Neutrinos, being quantum entities, exist in a superposition of flavor states. This means that a neutrino can exist simultaneously as an electron, muon, and tau neutrino, with each flavor having a certain probability associated with it.

Neutrino oscillation is driven by the mass differences between the three flavors. As neutrinos travel through space, their flavor composition changes, resulting in a fascinating interplay of the different flavors. This discovery, made possible through groundbreaking experiments, has revolutionized our understanding of neutrinos and has led to the realization that neutrinos have mass, albeit extremely tiny.

The implications of neutrino oscillation are significant for both theoretical and experimental particle physics. By studying these flavor changes, scientists can gain valuable insights into the properties of neutrinos, such as their masses and mixing angles. Moreover, neutrino oscillation has profound implications for our understanding of the cosmic balance between matter and antimatter, as well as the evolution of the universe.

Neutrino flavor states form the backbone of neutrino physics, providing a framework to describe the behavior and interactions of these elusive particles. Through meticulous experiments and theoretical advancements, scientists continue to unravel the mysteries surrounding neutrinos, contributing to our knowledge of the fundamental building blocks of the universe.

Whether you are a particle physics enthusiast or simply curious about the wonders of the universe, exploring the concept of neutrino flavor states will open doors to a captivating world where particles can morph and change their identity. Join us on this incredible journey as we dive deeper into the realm of neutrino physics, from basics to advanced concepts.

The Pontecorvo-Maki-Nakagawa-Sakata (PMNS) Matrix

The Pontecorvo-Maki-Nakagawa-Sakata (PMNS) matrix is a fundamental concept in the field of particle physics, specifically in the study of neutrinos. In this subchapter, we will explore the significance and applications of the PMNS matrix, shedding light on its role in understanding the behavior and properties of these elusive particles.

Neutrinos, often referred to as "ghost particles," are one of the most abundant yet least understood particles in the universe. They are electrically neutral and interact only through the weak nuclear force, making them incredibly challenging to detect and study. However, the PMNS matrix provides a powerful framework for unraveling the mysteries of neutrinos.

The PMNS matrix is named after Ziro Maki, Masami Nakagawa, and Shoichi Sakata, who, in collaboration with an Italian physicist Bruno Pontecorvo, proposed the mathematical formalism in 1962. It describes the relationship between the three known neutrino flavors (electron, muon, and tau) and their corresponding mass states. The matrix elements connect the flavor eigenstates to the mass eigenstates, providing insight into the phenomenon of neutrino oscillation.

Neutrino oscillation refers to the phenomenon where neutrinos change from one flavor to another as they travel through space. This discovery, which was awarded the Nobel Prize in Physics in 2015, revolutionized our understanding of neutrinos and solidified the importance of the PMNS matrix in the field of particle physics.

The PMNS matrix is a 3x3 unitary matrix, meaning that it has three rows and three columns with complex numbers as its elements. To understand neutrino oscillation, we need to examine the matrix elements and their corresponding phases. These phases play a crucial role in determining the probabilities of neutrinos transitioning between different flavors.

The PMNS matrix has far-reaching implications, not only in understanding the properties of neutrinos but also in addressing fundamental questions in particle physics. For instance, it has implications for the search for physics beyond the Standard Model, such as the existence of sterile neutrinos or the violation of CP symmetry.

In conclusion, the PMNS matrix is a fundamental concept in neutrino physics, providing the mathematical framework to understand neutrino oscillation and unravel the properties of these mysterious particles. Its significance extends beyond the field of particle physics, impacting our understanding of the universe's fundamental building blocks. By studying the PMNS matrix, we move closer to unraveling the secrets of neutrinos and opening doors to new realms of knowledge in particle physics.

Neutrino Oscillation Experiments

In the fascinating world of particle physics, one of the most intriguing phenomena to study is neutrino oscillation. Neutrinos, often referred to as the "ghost particles" of the universe, have the peculiar property of changing from one type to another as they travel through space. This transformation, known as neutrino oscillation, has revolutionized our understanding of these elusive particles and has opened up new avenues for scientific exploration.

Neutrino oscillation experiments have played a pivotal role in unraveling the mysteries surrounding these particles. These experiments involve studying the behavior of neutrinos produced in various sources, such as the Sun, nuclear reactors, or cosmic rays, and detecting them using specialized detectors. By carefully analyzing the data collected from these experiments, scientists have been able to elucidate the fundamental properties of neutrinos and shed light on their role in the cosmic processes.

The discovery of neutrino oscillation has fundamentally challenged the long-held notion that neutrinos are massless particles. It suggests that neutrinos have finite masses and that they can transition between different flavors - electron, muon, and tau neutrinos - as they propagate through space. This groundbreaking revelation has revolutionized our understanding of particle physics and has led to the development of the Standard Model of particle physics, which now incorporates neutrino oscillation.

Neutrino oscillation experiments have employed various innovative techniques to observe and measure these elusive particles. One such experiment is the Super-Kamiokande detector in Japan, which is a massive underground tank filled with ultra-pure water and surrounded by sensitive light detectors. This experiment has provided crucial evidence for neutrino oscillation by detecting neutrinos from cosmic rays and neutrinos produced in the Earth's atmosphere.

Other experiments, such as the Sudbury Neutrino Observatory (SNO) in Canada and the KamLAND experiment in Japan, have also made significant contributions to the field. The SNO experiment observed neutrinos emitted by the Sun and confirmed the existence of neutrino oscillation, while KamLAND detected anti-neutrinos emitted by nuclear reactors, further confirming the phenomenon.

Neutrino oscillation experiments continue to be at the forefront of particle physics research, with ongoing experiments like the Deep Underground Neutrino Experiment (DUNE) in the United States pushing the boundaries even further. These experiments aim to unravel the remaining mysteries surrounding neutrino oscillation, such as the precise measurement of neutrino masses and the determination of the so-called "CP-violation" phase, which could provide insights into why the universe is predominantly composed of matter rather than antimatter.

In conclusion, neutrino oscillation experiments have revolutionized our understanding of neutrinos and their role in the universe. These experiments have provided crucial evidence for the existence of neutrino oscillation and have opened up new avenues for scientific exploration. With ongoing research and advancements in technology, the study of neutrino oscillation promises to unlock even more profound insights into the fundamental nature of our universe.

Chapter 3: Neutrino Sources and Detection

Neutrino Sources: Solar, Atmospheric, and Supernovae

In the vast field of particle physics, few particles have captured the curiosity and fascination of scientists quite like neutrinos. These elusive particles, often referred to as "ghost particles," are electrically neutral and interact only weakly with matter, making them incredibly challenging to detect. However, their study has provided invaluable insights into the fundamental properties of the universe. In this subchapter, we will explore the three primary sources of neutrinos: the Sun, the Earth's atmosphere, and supernovae.

First and foremost, the Sun serves as an abundant source of neutrinos. Nuclear fusion reactions at its core generate a tremendous amount of energy, releasing vast numbers of neutrinos in the process. These solar neutrinos carry valuable information about the Sun's internal processes and have played a crucial role in confirming our understanding of how stars produce energy.

Moving on, the Earth's atmosphere also produces a significant number of neutrinos. High-energy cosmic rays from outer space continuously bombard the Earth's atmosphere, generating a cascade of secondary particles, including neutrinos. These atmospheric neutrinos provide scientists with a unique opportunity to study the properties and behavior of neutrinos, paving the way for advancements in our understanding of particle physics.

Finally, one of the most extraordinary events in the universe, a supernova explosion, produces an immense burst of neutrinos. When a massive star reaches the end of its life and undergoes a supernova, the gravitational collapse of its core releases an enormous amount of energy, creating a cataclysmic explosion. This explosion generates an intense flux of neutrinos, carrying vital information about the supernova's dynamics and the formation of neutron stars or black holes.

Studying these diverse sources of neutrinos has revolutionized our understanding of particle physics and the nature of the universe. Neutrinos have been instrumental in confirming the theory of solar fusion, providing evidence for the existence of neutrino oscillation (a phenomenon where neutrinos change their flavor as they travel through space), and offering insights into the inner workings of supernovae.

In conclusion, neutrinos are fascinating particles that have captivated the attention of scientists in the field of particle physics. Their sources, including the Sun, the Earth's atmosphere, and supernovae, offer unique opportunities for studying their properties and unlocking the mysteries of the universe. By delving into these sources, we can gain a deeper understanding of the fundamental nature of matter, energy, and the forces that govern our existence.

Neutrino Detection Techniques: Scintillation Detectors and Cherenkov Radiation

In the fascinating world of particle physics, the study of neutrinos holds a special place. These elusive particles, which are abundant in the universe, interact weakly with matter, making their detection a challenging task. However, scientists have developed ingenious techniques to unravel the mysteries of neutrinos. Two such techniques are scintillation detectors and the observation of Cherenkov radiation.

Scintillation detectors utilize the energy transfer that occurs when a neutrino interacts with a material. This interaction produces charged particles that, upon passing through a scintillating material, excite its atoms. As the atoms return to their ground state, they emit light in the form of flashes or scintillation. Photomultiplier tubes surrounding the scintillator convert these flashes into electrical signals that can be measured and analyzed. Scintillation detectors are widely used due to their high sensitivity, relatively low cost, and ability to detect neutrinos across a wide range of energies.

On the other hand, Cherenkov radiation is a phenomenon that occurs when a charged particle moves faster than the speed of light in a medium. Neutrinos rarely interact with matter, but occasionally, highly energetic neutrinos can collide with atomic nuclei or electrons in a medium. These collisions create charged particles that move faster than the speed of light in that medium, emitting a faint bluish glow known as Cherenkov radiation. This radiation can be detected using specialized photomultiplier tubes, which capture the light and convert it into an electrical signal for analysis.

Both scintillation detectors and Cherenkov radiation detection techniques have their unique advantages and applications. Scintillation detectors are particularly useful for detecting low-energy neutrinos and have been widely employed in underground experiments, such as those studying solar neutrinos or neutrinos from nuclear reactors. Cherenkov radiation, on the other hand, is primarily used to detect high-energy neutrinos, such as those produced in cosmic ray interactions with the Earth's atmosphere or in astrophysical sources.

Understanding the properties and behavior of neutrinos is crucial for advancing our knowledge of the universe. By employing innovative techniques like scintillation detectors and Cherenkov radiation detection, scientists can overcome the challenges posed by neutrinos' weak interactions and shed light on their mysterious nature. These methods have revolutionized the field of neutrino physics and continue to provide valuable insights into the fundamental building blocks of our universe.

Whether you are a particle physicist or simply curious about the wonders of the cosmos, exploring the intricacies of neutrino detection techniques will open doors to a world of scientific discovery and fascination.

Neutrino Observatories: IceCube, Super-Kamiokande, and Others

In the fascinating world of particle physics, neutrinos play a unique and mysterious role. These elusive particles are abundant in the universe, yet they interact very weakly with matter, making them extremely difficult to detect. Neutrino observatories have been instrumental in unraveling the secrets of these enigmatic particles, and in this subchapter, we will explore two prominent examples: IceCube and Super-Kamiokande, along with other notable neutrino observatories.

IceCube, located at the South Pole, is the world's largest neutrino detector. Buried deep beneath the ice, it consists of thousands of optical sensors arranged in a grid-like pattern. When a neutrino interacts with the ice, it produces a secondary particle called a muon. As the muon moves through the ice, it emits a faint blue light, known as Cherenkov radiation, which is detected by the sensors. By analyzing the arrival time and direction of these light signals, scientists can determine the energy and origin of the neutrinos. IceCube has provided valuable insights into the high-energy neutrino sources, such as supernovae, gamma-ray bursts, and even cosmic rays from distant galaxies.

Super-Kamiokande, situated in Japan, is another groundbreaking neutrino observatory. Unlike IceCube, Super-Kamiokande is a water-based detector. It consists of a massive tank filled with ultrapure water and lined with sensitive photomultiplier tubes. When a neutrino collides with a water molecule, it produces a charged particle, which emits Cherenkov radiation. The photomultiplier tubes capture these light signals, enabling scientists to reconstruct the direction and energy of the incoming neutrinos. Super-Kamiokande has made significant contributions to the study of solar neutrinos, atmospheric neutrinos, and neutrino oscillations, leading to the discovery that neutrinos have mass.

Apart from IceCube and Super-Kamiokande, several other neutrino observatories have added to our understanding of these elusive particles. ANTARES, located deep in the Mediterranean Sea, and Borexino, nestled beneath the Italian Gran Sasso mountain, are two notable examples. Each observatory utilizes different detection techniques, providing complementary data for comprehensive neutrino research.

The study of neutrinos has revolutionized our understanding of the universe, from the inner workings of stars to the fundamental laws of particle physics. Neutrino observatories like IceCube, Super-Kamiokande, and others continue to push the boundaries of our knowledge, unlocking the mysteries of these ghostly particles. Whether you are a particle physics enthusiast or simply curious about the wonders of the universe, exploring the world of neutrino observatories will undoubtedly ignite your curiosity and expand your understanding of this intriguing field.

Chapter 4: Neutrino Mass and Mixing

Neutrino Mass Hierarchy

In the fascinating realm of particle physics, the study of neutrinos has opened up a whole new frontier of knowledge. Neutrinos, often called "ghost particles," are elusive and mysterious, yet they play a crucial role in understanding the fundamental properties of the universe. One of the most intriguing aspects of neutrinos is their mass hierarchy, which has captivated the scientific community for decades.

Neutrinos are elementary particles that interact only weakly with matter, making them extremely difficult to detect. They come in three flavors: electron, muon, and tau, and each flavor is associated with a different particle in the Standard Model of particle physics. The discovery that neutrinos can change their flavor during their journey, known as neutrino oscillation, was a groundbreaking revelation that hinted at the existence of neutrino mass.

Determining the hierarchy of neutrino masses has been a long-standing challenge. Scientists have proposed two possible hierarchies: the normal hierarchy, where the mass of the electron neutrino is the smallest, followed by the muon neutrino and tau neutrino, and the inverted hierarchy, where the mass of the tau neutrino is the smallest. Understanding the neutrino mass hierarchy is crucial for unraveling the mysteries associated with neutrino oscillation and could provide insights into the fundamental nature of matter and the evolution of the universe.

Experimental efforts to determine the neutrino mass hierarchy have been underway for years. One such approach is the study of neutrino oscillation patterns using powerful neutrino detectors located deep underground. These experiments involve firing a beam of neutrinos and observing the changes in flavor as they travel through matter. By carefully analyzing the observed oscillation patterns, scientists hope to unravel the mass hierarchy puzzle.

The discovery of the neutrino mass hierarchy could have far-reaching implications. It could shed light on the phenomenon of matter-antimatter asymmetry, one of the greatest mysteries in physics. It could also provide insights into the nature of dark matter and the evolution of the universe. Moreover, understanding neutrino masses could have implications for the stability of the sun and other astrophysical phenomena.

In conclusion, the study of neutrino mass hierarchy is a captivating and complex field of research within particle physics. It is an area that holds immense potential for advancing our understanding of the fundamental building blocks of the universe. As scientists continue to explore this intriguing topic, the answers they uncover may revolutionize our understanding of the cosmos and pave the way for exciting new discoveries.

Absolute Neutrino Mass Measurements

Neutrinos, often referred to as the "ghost particles" of the universe, have captivated the attention of scientists for decades. These elusive particles possess astonishing properties that challenge our understanding of the fundamental laws of physics. One of the most intriguing aspects of neutrinos is their mass, which has long been a subject of intense research and debate. In this subchapter, we delve into the fascinating world of absolute neutrino mass measurements, shedding light on the current state of knowledge in the field.

Neutrinos were initially believed to be massless, but groundbreaking experiments conducted in the late 20th century shattered this perception. The discovery of neutrino oscillations, which occurs when neutrinos change between different flavors (electron, muon, and tau), provided the first evidence that neutrinos have non-zero masses. However, the exact values of these masses remain unknown, posing a significant challenge for particle physicists.

There are two primary methods employed to determine the absolute masses of neutrinos: direct and indirect measurements. Direct measurements involve experiments aimed at capturing and analyzing neutrinos themselves, while indirect measurements rely on cosmological observations and the study of large-scale structures in the universe.

Direct measurements depend on the phenomenon of beta decay, which involves the emission of an electron or positron by a radioactive nucleus. By precisely measuring the energy distribution of the emitted particles, scientists can infer the mass of the neutrinos involved in the process. Various experiments, such as the Karlsruhe Tritium Neutrino (KATRIN) experiment, are pushing the limits of sensitivity to detect the tiny effects of neutrino masses in beta decay processes.

On the other hand, indirect measurements exploit the effects of neutrino masses on the cosmic microwave background (CMB) radiation, the relic radiation from the early universe. By analyzing the CMB power spectrum and the large-scale structure of the universe, researchers can constrain the sum of the masses of all three neutrino flavors. These measurements, combined with data from other cosmological observations, provide valuable insights into the absolute masses of neutrinos.

While significant progress has been made in recent years, determining the precise values of neutrino masses still presents a major challenge. The masses of neutrinos are exceptionally small, making them extraordinarily difficult to measure accurately. However, advancements in technology, such as improved detectors and more sensitive experiments, offer hope for future breakthroughs in this field.

In conclusion, absolute neutrino mass measurements represent a crucial frontier in particle physics. Understanding the masses of neutrinos is not only essential for completing the Standard Model of particle physics but also has profound implications for cosmology and the nature of the universe. Continued research in this area will undoubtedly shed new light on the mysterious properties of these ghostly particles and deepen our understanding of the fundamental fabric of reality.

Leptogenesis and Neutrino Mass

In the exciting realm of particle physics, the study of neutrinos has become a captivating and rapidly evolving field. Neutrinos, often referred to as the "ghost particles" of the universe, are fascinating subatomic particles that are electrically neutral and exhibit extremely weak interactions with matter. They are produced in various astrophysical and terrestrial processes, and their properties have perplexed scientists for decades. This subchapter explores the intriguing connection between leptogenesis and neutrino mass and sheds light on this intricate relationship.

Leptogenesis is a theoretical framework that seeks to explain the observed matter-antimatter asymmetry in the universe. It proposes that the early universe was dominated by a primordial soup of particles, including neutrinos and their antiparticles. Through a process known as leptonic CP violation, a subtle difference in the behavior of neutrinos and antineutrinos can arise, leading to an excess of matter over antimatter. This excess is then responsible for the existence of our matter-dominated universe.

Furthermore, leptogenesis is closely linked to the phenomenon of neutrino mass. While neutrinos were initially believed to be massless, numerous experimental observations have confirmed that they do possess a small but finite mass. The discovery of neutrino oscillations, where neutrinos change their flavor as they propagate through space, was a groundbreaking revelation that provided strong evidence for neutrino mass.

This subchapter delves into the theoretical mechanisms behind neutrino mass generation and explores the implications for leptogenesis. One of the leading proposals is the seesaw mechanism, which postulates the existence of heavy right-handed neutrinos. These right-handed neutrinos have large masses and interact with the lighter left-handed neutrinos, leading to a suppressed overall neutrino mass scale. This mechanism not only provides a compelling explanation for the smallness of neutrino masses but also offers a natural framework for leptogenesis to occur.

Understanding leptogenesis and neutrino mass is of profound importance as it sheds light on fundamental questions about the structure of the universe and its evolution. By unraveling the mysteries surrounding these ghostly particles, scientists hope to gain deeper insights into the fundamental laws of nature and the origins of matter itself.

Whether you are an aspiring physicist, a curious science enthusiast, or simply someone intrigued by the wonders of the universe, this subchapter will provide a comprehensive and accessible introduction to the captivating world of leptogenesis and neutrino mass. Join us as we embark on a journey through the fundamental concepts, theoretical models, and experimental discoveries that have shaped our understanding of these enigmatic particles.

Chapter 5: Neutrino Interactions with Matter

Charged Current and Neutral Current Interactions

In the realm of particle physics, the study of neutrinos holds a special place due to their intriguing properties and their role in shaping our understanding of the fundamental building blocks of the universe. Neutrinos, often referred to as ghostly particles, are electrically neutral and interact only weakly with matter. This unique characteristic makes them challenging to detect and study, but it also provides a fascinating avenue for exploring the mysteries of the subatomic world.

One of the key concepts in neutrino physics is understanding the different types of interactions that neutrinos can undergo. Two major categories of interactions are charged current and neutral current interactions. These interactions play a crucial role in the behavior of neutrinos and shed light on their properties.

Charged current interactions involve the exchange of a charged W boson, which transfers energy and momentum between a neutrino and a target particle. This interaction can result in the transformation of a neutrino of one flavor into another. For example, an electron neutrino can interact with a proton, producing a neutron and a positron. This process provides valuable information about the mixing of neutrino flavors and the phenomenon known as neutrino oscillation.

On the other hand, neutral current interactions occur when a neutrino interacts with a target particle via the exchange of a neutral Z boson. In this case, the neutrino does not change its flavor but can still transfer energy and momentum. Neutral current interactions contribute to the overall understanding of neutrino properties, such as their cross-sections and scattering angles.

Studying charged current and neutral current interactions is crucial for various fields of research, including astrophysics, cosmology, and particle physics. Neutrinos are produced in various astrophysical sources, such as the sun, supernovae, and cosmic rays. By studying the interactions of neutrinos from these sources, scientists can gain insights into the processes occurring within these celestial objects.

In particle physics experiments, charged current and neutral current interactions are carefully measured to determine the properties of neutrinos, such as their masses, mixing angles, and flavor compositions. These measurements contribute to our understanding of the Standard Model of particle physics and can provide hints towards new physics beyond the known framework.

In summary, charged current and neutral current interactions are fundamental concepts in the study of neutrinos. Understanding these interactions helps unravel the mysteries of neutrino properties and their role in the universe. From the behavior of neutrinos in astrophysical sources to their measurements in particle physics experiments, charged current and neutral current interactions offer a gateway to unlocking the secrets of the subatomic world.

Neutrino-Nucleus Scattering

Neutrinos are fascinating and elusive particles that have captivated the imagination of physicists for decades. In this subchapter, we will delve into the intricacies of neutrino-nucleus scattering, a fundamental process in particle physics that sheds light on the nature of neutrinos and their interactions with matter.

Neutrino-nucleus scattering occurs when a neutrino, one of the most abundant yet elusive particles in the universe, interacts with a nucleus. This interaction provides valuable insights into the properties of neutrinos, such as their mass, flavor, and oscillation behavior. It also allows us to study the structure of atomic nuclei and the fundamental forces that govern their interactions with neutrinos.

To understand neutrino-nucleus scattering, we must first grasp the basics of neutrinos. Neutrinos are subatomic particles that possess a tiny mass and no electric charge. They come in three different flavors – electron, muon, and tau – and can oscillate or transform between these flavors as they propagate through space. This phenomenon is known as neutrino oscillation and has revolutionized our understanding of particle physics.

When a neutrino interacts with a nucleus, it can either scatter off the nucleus without changing its flavor or undergo a process called charged-current (CC) interaction, where it exchanges a W boson with a nucleus. In the latter case, the neutrino can change its flavor, providing crucial evidence for neutrino oscillation.

Neutrino-nucleus scattering experiments are conducted using sophisticated detectors, such as liquid argon time projection chambers or scintillator-based detectors. These detectors are designed to capture the elusive signals produced when neutrinos interact with atomic nuclei. By carefully analyzing these signals, physicists can extract valuable information about the properties of neutrinos, such as their energy, momentum, and interaction cross-sections.

Understanding neutrino-nucleus scattering is crucial for a wide range of scientific endeavors. It has important implications for astrophysics, as neutrinos are produced in abundance during high-energy cosmic events, such as supernovae. By studying neutrino-nucleus scattering, scientists can gain insights into the inner workings of these cataclysmic events and decipher the mysteries of the universe.

In summary, neutrino-nucleus scattering is a fascinating process that allows us to probe the properties of neutrinos and the structure of atomic nuclei. It is a fundamental aspect of particle physics and has far-reaching implications for our understanding of the universe. By unraveling the mysteries of neutrino-nucleus scattering, scientists are paving the way for groundbreaking discoveries in the realm of particle physics and astrophysics.

Neutrino-Electron Scattering

In the fascinating world of particle physics, one of the most intriguing phenomena is neutrino-electron scattering. This subchapter aims to unravel the mysteries behind this intriguing interaction, exploring its significance and shedding light on its relevance in the field of neutrino physics.

Neutrinos are elusive particles that interact weakly with matter, making them notoriously difficult to detect and study. However, their interactions with electrons provide valuable insights into their properties and behavior. Neutrino-electron scattering occurs when a neutrino interacts with an electron, resulting in a scattered electron and a modified neutrino.

The study of neutrino-electron scattering has proven to be crucial in understanding the fundamental properties of neutrinos. By examining the energy and angle of the scattered electron, physicists can deduce valuable information about the neutrino's momentum and energy. This, in turn, allows researchers to investigate the neutrino's mass, flavor, and oscillation patterns.

One of the fundamental aspects of neutrino-electron scattering is its connection to the weak force. As one of the four fundamental forces in nature, the weak force governs the interactions of subatomic particles. Neutrinos, being weakly interacting particles, are primarily affected by this force. By studying neutrino-electron scattering, scientists can probe the underlying mechanisms of the weak force, providing insights into the fundamental nature of the universe.

Neutrino-electron scattering experiments have played a pivotal role in confirming the existence of neutrinos and their flavor oscillations. Through these experiments, physicists have gathered evidence that neutrinos can change from one flavor to another, challenging the conventional understanding of particle physics and opening up new avenues of research.

Moreover, neutrino-electron scattering has practical applications beyond fundamental research. Understanding this interaction is crucial for the development of detectors that can accurately measure and identify neutrinos. Such detectors are essential for studying neutrinos from various sources, including the Sun, cosmic rays, and even man-made neutrino beams.

In conclusion, neutrino-electron scattering is a captivating aspect of particle physics that offers valuable insights into the nature of neutrinos and the weak force. Its study has revolutionized our understanding of neutrinos and their oscillations, leading to groundbreaking discoveries in the field. With its significance ranging from fundamental research to practical applications, this subchapter serves as a gateway to the captivating world of neutrino physics for readers of all backgrounds.

Chapter 6: Neutrino Phenomenology

Neutrino Physics Beyond the Standard Model

The world of particle physics is an ever-evolving field, constantly pushing the boundaries of our knowledge and understanding of the fundamental building blocks of the universe. Neutrinos, elusive and mysterious particles, hold a special place in this exciting realm. In this subchapter, we delve into the intriguing world of neutrino physics beyond the Standard Model, exploring the cutting-edge research and advanced concepts that continue to captivate scientists and enthusiasts alike.

The Standard Model of particle physics has been remarkably successful in explaining the behavior and interactions of known particles. However, it falls short when it comes to understanding the nature of neutrinos. Neutrinos are known to possess intriguing properties, such as their ability to oscillate between different flavors (electron, muon, and tau). This phenomenon implies that neutrinos have mass, which conflicts with the initial assumption of the Standard Model.

To unravel these mysteries, researchers have proposed several extensions to the Standard Model. One such concept is the seesaw mechanism, which offers a compelling explanation for the tiny masses of neutrinos. This theory suggests the existence of new, heavy particles that interact with neutrinos, providing a mechanism for the observed mass hierarchy. Exploring the seesaw mechanism has become a major focus of experimental and theoretical investigations in neutrino physics.

Another fascinating avenue of research is the quest for sterile neutrinos. Unlike the three known flavors, sterile neutrinos do not interact via the weak nuclear force, making them even more challenging to detect. The existence of sterile neutrinos could have profound implications for our understanding of the universe, including their potential role in dark matter and the matter-antimatter asymmetry conundrum.

Moreover, the search for neutrinoless double-beta decay, a process that violates lepton number conservation, has gained significant attention. The observation of this decay would provide crucial insights into the nature of neutrinos and could shed light on why matter dominates over antimatter in the universe.

As we embark on this journey into neutrino physics beyond the Standard Model, it is essential to recognize the immense technological advancements that have made these investigations possible. Large-scale experiments like the Super-Kamiokande, IceCube, and DUNE are pushing the boundaries of neutrino detection, enhancing our ability to study neutrinos in unprecedented detail.

In conclusion, the subchapter on Neutrino Physics Beyond the Standard Model provides a glimpse into the cutting-edge research and advanced concepts that are shaping our understanding of neutrinos. From the seesaw mechanism to sterile neutrinos and neutrinoless double-beta decay, these explorations have the potential to revolutionize our knowledge of the universe and bring us closer to solving some of its deepest mysteries. Whether you are a particle physics enthusiast or simply curious about the frontiers of science, this subchapter promises to take you on an exhilarating journey into the captivating world of neutrino physics.

Neutrinoless Double Beta Decay

In the fascinating world of particle physics, one phenomenon that has captured the attention of scientists worldwide is neutrinoless double beta decay. This subatomic process holds the key to unraveling the mysterious properties of neutrinos, the elusive particles that can pass through matter without any interaction. In this chapter, we will delve into the intricacies of neutrinoless double beta decay, exploring its significance and the implications it holds for our understanding of the universe.

Neutrinoless double beta decay refers to a rare nuclear decay process in which two neutrons within an atomic nucleus simultaneously transform into two protons, emitting only electrons (beta particles) and no neutrinos. This decay, if observed, would provide striking evidence for the existence of a phenomenon called lepton number violation, a fundamental principle in particle physics. The observation of neutrinoless double beta decay would also confirm that neutrinos are their own antiparticles, a property known as Majorana nature.

The implications of neutrinoless double beta decay extend beyond the realm of particle physics. It could shed light on the fundamental question of why there is more matter than antimatter in the universe, a phenomenon known as the matter-antimatter asymmetry. Additionally, it could help determine the absolute mass scale of neutrinos, which is crucial for understanding their role in the evolution of the cosmos and the formation of galaxies.

Efforts to detect neutrinoless double beta decay are currently underway in various experiments around the world. These experiments involve the use of sophisticated detectors, such as cryogenic devices and scintillators, to identify the telltale signatures of the decay process. Furthermore, the construction of large-scale experiments, such as the upcoming nEXO and LEGEND projects, aims to enhance the sensitivity and reach of neutrinoless double beta decay searches.

While the detection of neutrinoless double beta decay remains an ongoing challenge, its potential discovery would mark a major milestone in our understanding of the fundamental building blocks of the universe. It would not only confirm the existence of lepton number violation and the Majorana nature of neutrinos but also pave the way for further breakthroughs in particle physics and cosmology.

In conclusion, neutrinoless double beta decay is a captivating topic in the field of particle physics. Its investigation holds promise for unraveling the mysteries surrounding neutrinos and their role in the universe. As scientists continue to push the boundaries of experimental techniques and technology, we eagerly await the day when neutrinoless double beta decay is finally observed, providing us with new insights into the fundamental nature of our universe.

Neutrino Astrophysics: Supernovae and Neutrino Astronomy

In the vast expanse of the universe, countless stars are born, live out their lives, and eventually meet their demise in spectacular explosions known as supernovae. These cataclysmic events release an enormous amount of energy and generate a myriad of particles, including the elusive neutrinos. In the subchapter of "A Beginner's Guide to Neutrino Physics: From Basics to Advanced Concepts" titled "Neutrino Astrophysics: Supernovae and Neutrino Astronomy," we delve into the fascinating world of neutrinos and their role in understanding the universe.

Addressed to a wide audience, including enthusiasts of particle physics, this subchapter provides a comprehensive overview of the field of neutrino astrophysics. Neutrinos, the ghostly particles that interact weakly with matter, play a crucial role in unraveling the mysteries of supernovae and expanding our understanding of the cosmos.

Supernovae, the explosive deaths of massive stars, emit an enormous burst of neutrinos. These neutrinos, produced during the core collapse and subsequent explosion, carry vital information about the physical processes occurring inside the star. By studying the neutrinos emitted from a supernova, scientists can gain insights into the dynamics of the explosion, the formation of neutron stars or black holes, and the synthesis of heavy elements.

This subchapter explores the methods used in neutrino astronomy to detect and study these elusive particles emitted from supernovae. From large-scale underground detectors, such as Super-Kamiokande and IceCube, to space-based observatories like the future DUNE detector, we discuss the different techniques employed to capture neutrinos and extract valuable data.

Furthermore, the subchapter delves into the exciting discoveries made in neutrino astrophysics, including the detection of neutrinos from the famous Supernova 1987A. This groundbreaking event provided substantial evidence for the core-collapse mechanism of supernovae and confirmed the predictions of stellar evolution models.

The subchapter also touches upon the ongoing and future experiments aimed at detecting neutrinos from supernovae in our galaxy and beyond. These endeavors hold the promise of shedding light on numerous astrophysical phenomena, such as the formation of neutron stars, the origin of cosmic rays, and the evolution of galaxies.

By presenting the concepts and methods of neutrino astrophysics in a beginner-friendly manner, this subchapter aims to captivate the interests of both particle physics enthusiasts and anyone intrigued by the wonders of the universe. Through the study of neutrinos emitted from supernovae, we embark on a journey to unravel the mysteries of the cosmos, expanding our horizons and deepening our understanding of the fundamental laws that govern our universe.

Chapter 7: Neutrino Experiments and Future Prospects

Current Neutrino Experiments: Daya Bay, T2K, and NOvA

Neutrino physics is an exciting and rapidly evolving field within particle physics, offering unique insights into the fundamental building blocks of our universe. In this subchapter, we will explore three of the most prominent neutrino experiments: Daya Bay, T2K, and NOvA. These experiments are at the forefront of neutrino research and have significantly contributed to our understanding of these elusive particles.

The Daya Bay experiment, located in southern China, aims to measure a phenomenon known as neutrino oscillation. Neutrinos come in three flavors: electron, muon, and tau. Through a process called oscillation, neutrinos can change from one flavor to another as they travel through space. Daya Bay investigates this phenomenon by studying the disappearance of electron antineutrinos emitted from nuclear reactors. By carefully measuring the rate at which these antineutrinos vanish, researchers can determine the mixing angles and mass differences between the neutrino flavors.

Moving on to T2K, the Tokai to Kamioka experiment, which takes place in Japan, focuses on another aspect of neutrino oscillation: neutrino appearance. T2K produces a beam of muon neutrinos at the J-PARC accelerator and directs it towards the Super-Kamiokande detector, located 295 kilometers away. By analyzing the interactions of the neutrinos in the detector, scientists can study the phenomenon of neutrino oscillation and gain insights into the properties of neutrinos, such as their masses and mixing angles.

Lastly, the NOvA experiment, situated in the United States, is designed to investigate the same phenomenon as T2K but with a different approach. NOvA uses two detectors: one located at Fermilab near Chicago and another in Ash River, Minnesota, approximately 810 kilometers away. Similar to T2K, NOvA sends a beam of muon neutrinos through the Earth's crust and measures the oscillation pattern at the distant detector. By comparing the data from both detectors, researchers can precisely determine the neutrino oscillation parameters.

These experiments have significantly contributed to our current understanding of neutrinos. They have confirmed the existence of neutrino oscillation and shed light on the properties of these elusive particles. Their findings have challenged our existing theories and have the potential to revolutionize our understanding of the universe at its most fundamental level.

As a beginner in the field of particle physics, exploring the intricacies of neutrino experiments like Daya Bay, T2K, and NOvA can be a fascinating journey. These experiments not only push the boundaries of scientific knowledge but also have the potential to reshape our understanding of the universe. By delving into the details of these experiments, you can gain a deeper appreciation for the complex nature of neutrinos and the cutting-edge research being conducted to unravel their mysteries. So, join us as we embark on this captivating exploration of neutrino physics and the experiments that are shaping the future of particle physics.

Future Neutrino Experiments: DUNE, Hyper-Kamiokande, and JUNO

In recent years, neutrino physics has emerged as a captivating field within the domain of particle physics. Neutrinos, often referred to as "ghost particles," are among the most elusive and mysterious particles in the universe. They possess intriguing properties, such as their ability to oscillate between different flavors, making them fascinating subjects of scientific study. In this subchapter, we will explore three future neutrino experiments: DUNE, Hyper-Kamiokande, and JUNO, which hold great promise for unraveling the mysteries surrounding these enigmatic particles.

First on our list is the Deep Underground Neutrino Experiment (DUNE), a groundbreaking international collaboration set to be conducted in the United States. DUNE aims to investigate neutrino oscillations with unprecedented precision by utilizing a massive liquid argon detector located deep underground. This ambitious experiment will help elucidate the neutrino mass hierarchy, determine whether neutrinos violate the fundamental symmetry known as CP, and potentially uncover new physics beyond the Standard Model.

Next, we have Hyper-Kamiokande, an upgrade of the renowned Super-Kamiokande experiment in Japan. Hyper-Kamiokande is set to be the world's largest neutrino detector, comprising a colossal water tank surrounded by highly sensitive light sensors. This experiment will focus on measuring neutrino oscillations, precisely determining neutrino properties, and exploring neutrinos' role in the evolution of the universe. Hyper-Kamiokande's enhanced capabilities will enable scientists to delve deeper into the mysteries of neutrino physics.

Lastly, we introduce JUNO (Jiangmen Underground Neutrino Observatory), a unique experiment taking place in China. JUNO plans to employ a massive liquid scintillator detector to investigate neutrinos emitted from a nearby nuclear power plant. By precisely measuring the energy spectra and oscillation behavior of these reactor neutrinos, JUNO aims to address fundamental questions, including the neutrino mass ordering and the existence of sterile neutrinos. This experiment will contribute significantly to our understanding of neutrino properties and their role in astrophysical phenomena.

These future neutrino experiments hold immense potential to revolutionize our understanding of the universe at its most fundamental level. They will shed light on the mysterious properties of neutrinos and their implications for particle physics, astrophysics, and cosmology. These endeavors are not only of interest to particle physicists but also to a broader audience who seeks to comprehend the fundamental building blocks of our universe. As we embark on these groundbreaking experiments, we can anticipate remarkable discoveries and a deeper understanding of the enigmatic neutrinos that permeate our world.

Neutrino Physics at Colliders: The Long-Baseline Neutrino Facility (LBNF)

In the fascinating realm of particle physics, one of the most intriguing and elusive particles is the neutrino. Being the most abundant yet least understood particle in the universe, neutrinos hold the key to unraveling the mysteries of the cosmos. To shed light on their properties and behaviors, scientists have developed cutting-edge facilities such as the Long-Baseline Neutrino Facility (LBNF).

The LBNF is a state-of-the-art experimental setup designed to study neutrinos in a controlled and precise manner. It utilizes powerful particle colliders to create intense beams of neutrinos and then detects and analyzes the interactions of these particles with matter. This facility represents a remarkable achievement in the field of particle physics, providing scientists with unprecedented opportunities to unravel the secrets of neutrinos.

One of the primary goals of the LBNF is to investigate neutrino oscillations. Neutrinos come in three different types, or flavors: electron, muon, and tau. However, as they travel through space, neutrinos can spontaneously change from one flavor to another. This phenomenon, known as neutrino oscillation, implies that neutrinos have mass, a discovery that revolutionized our understanding of particle physics. By studying neutrino oscillations at the LBNF, scientists hope to gain deeper insights into the fundamental properties of these mysterious particles.

Another crucial aspect of the LBNF is its long-baseline feature. This means that the neutrino beams generated by the collider are directed to travel over long distances, often spanning hundreds of kilometers. By measuring the neutrino interactions at different distances, researchers are able to investigate how neutrinos evolve and change over time, further enhancing our understanding of their behavior.

The LBNF also plays a vital role in exploring the asymmetry between matter and antimatter in the universe. This phenomenon, called CP violation, might provide the missing link to understanding why the universe is predominantly composed of matter. By studying neutrinos at the LBNF, scientists aim to uncover the secrets behind this intriguing imbalance and shed light on the early moments of the universe's formation.

In conclusion, the Long-Baseline Neutrino Facility (LBNF) represents a groundbreaking tool in the field of neutrino physics. By utilizing advanced particle colliders, this facility enables scientists to study neutrinos in a controlled environment and explore their fundamental properties and behaviors. With its focus on neutrino oscillations, long-baseline observations, and matter-antimatter asymmetries, the LBNF offers a unique opportunity to push the boundaries of particle physics and deepen our understanding of the universe. Whether you are a beginner or an expert in the field, the LBNF's pursuit of neutrino physics opens up a world of knowledge and excitement for everyone interested in the fascinating realm of particle physics.

Chapter 8: Applications of Neutrino Physics

Neutrinos and Particle Astrophysics

In the vast landscape of particle physics, neutrinos have emerged as intriguing and elusive entities. These tiny, neutral particles are abundant in the universe, yet they interact weakly with matter, making them notoriously difficult to detect. This subchapter delves into the fascinating realm of neutrinos and their role in particle astrophysics, shedding light on their properties, origins, and their significance in understanding the cosmos.

Neutrinos, often referred to as "ghost particles," are elementary particles that belong to the lepton family, along with electrons and their heavier counterparts, the muons and taus. Unlike charged particles, neutrinos have no electric charge, and their masses are incredibly small, which has made their detection and study challenging for scientists.

The study of neutrinos has led to remarkable discoveries and groundbreaking insights in particle astrophysics. Neutrinos are produced in various astrophysical processes, such as nuclear reactions in the Sun, supernovae explosions, and high-energy cosmic ray interactions. These elusive particles carry valuable information about the sources and mechanisms of these astrophysical phenomena.

One of the key achievements in neutrino physics was the confirmation of neutrino oscillations, which established that neutrinos possess mass and can transform between different flavors (electron, muon, and tau) as they propagate through space. This groundbreaking discovery unlocked a new avenue for exploring the properties of neutrinos and their impact on the universe.

Particle astrophysics relies on the detection of neutrinos to unveil the mysteries of the cosmos. Neutrino observatories, such as IceCube at the South Pole and Super-Kamiokande in Japan, are designed to detect high-energy neutrinos from astrophysical sources. By studying the properties of these neutrinos, scientists can gain insights into the most extreme environments in the universe, such as black holes, neutron stars, and gamma-ray bursts.

Moreover, neutrinos play a crucial role in understanding the fundamental laws of physics. Their study provides valuable information about the Standard Model of particle physics, which describes the fundamental particles and their interactions. Neutrinos have the potential to challenge our current understanding of particle physics and provide clues to new physics beyond the Standard Model.

In conclusion, neutrinos and particle astrophysics offer a captivating journey into the depths of the universe. From their mysterious origins to their detection and study, neutrinos have revolutionized our understanding of particle physics and the cosmos. Unraveling the secrets of these ghostly particles holds the promise of unveiling new cosmic phenomena and advancing our knowledge of the fundamental laws governing the universe.

Neutrinos in Cosmology

The study of neutrinos in cosmology has revolutionized our understanding of the universe and its fundamental building blocks. Neutrinos, often called nature's "ghost particles," are elusive subatomic particles that have a negligible mass and interact very weakly with ordinary matter. They are produced in various astrophysical processes, such as nuclear reactions in the Sun, supernovae explosions, and even in the early moments of the universe's existence.

In the subatomic world, neutrinos play a crucial role in particle physics, but their significance goes beyond that. Neutrinos have a profound impact on cosmology, the science that explores the origin, evolution, and structure of the universe. These tiny particles, with their unique properties, have left an indelible imprint on the cosmic landscape, shaping the universe as we know it.

One of the most intriguing aspects of neutrinos in cosmology is their role in the early universe. During the first few seconds after the Big Bang, the universe was a seething soup of particles and radiation. Neutrinos, being weakly interacting, managed to escape this hot, dense environment, carrying valuable information about the early universe with them. By studying the cosmic neutrino background, scientists can gain insight into the conditions and dynamics of the universe during its infancy.

Furthermore, neutrinos have played a vital role in shaping the large-scale structure of the cosmos. As the universe expanded and cooled, neutrinos began to clump together under the influence of gravity. These neutrino "clumps" acted as seeds for the formation of galaxies and galaxy clusters. Understanding the role of neutrinos in structure formation is crucial for comprehending the cosmic web of galaxies we observe today.

Neutrinos also have implications for the fate of the universe. Their existence and properties have a direct connection to the total amount of matter in the cosmos and the rate of its expansion. By studying the behavior of neutrinos, scientists can make predictions about the ultimate destiny of our universe, whether it will continue expanding indefinitely or ultimately collapse upon itself.

In summary, neutrinos are not just fascinating particles in the realm of particle physics; they also play a vital role in cosmology. Their properties and behavior have shaped the universe from its earliest moments, leaving an imprint on the large-scale structure and influencing the fate of the cosmos. By unraveling the mysteries of neutrinos in cosmology, scientists are uncovering the secrets of the universe itself.

"A Beginner's Guide to Neutrino Physics: From Basics to Advanced Concepts" provides a comprehensive introduction to the world of neutrinos, including their significance in cosmology. Whether you are a particle physics enthusiast or someone curious about the mysteries of the universe, this book will take you on an exciting journey to understand the fundamental nature of neutrinos and their profound impact on the cosmos.

Neutrinos and Dark Matter

In the vast expanse of the universe, there are numerous mysteries that continue to perplex scientists and enthusiasts alike. Among these enigmatic phenomena are neutrinos and dark matter – two intriguing subjects that have captured the attention of particle physicists worldwide. In this subchapter, we will delve into the fascinating world of neutrinos and dark matter, shedding light on their significance in the field of particle physics.

Neutrinos, often referred to as "ghost particles," are elusive subatomic particles that travel at nearly the speed of light and possess no electric charge. They are constantly streaming through our bodies and the Earth, yet they interact so weakly with matter that they can effortlessly pass through solid objects, including planets and stars. Neutrinos come in three flavors – electron, muon, and tau – each associated with a corresponding charged lepton. The study of neutrinos has revolutionized our understanding of the universe, challenging existing theories and opening up new avenues of research.

Dark matter, on the other hand, is an invisible substance that permeates the cosmos and makes up a significant portion of the universe's mass. Although dark matter does not emit, absorb, or reflect light, its presence is inferred through its gravitational effects on visible matter. The search for dark matter has become one of the most pressing quests in modern physics, as its existence could hold the key to unraveling the mysteries of the universe. Scientists believe that dark matter plays a crucial role in the formation and structure of galaxies, influencing the distribution of visible matter and shaping the cosmic web.

The connection between neutrinos and dark matter lies in their shared properties of weak interaction. Neutrinos are the only known particles that interact solely through the weak force – the same force responsible for radioactive decay. Similarly, dark matter is hypothesized to interact weakly with ordinary matter, making it extremely challenging to detect. Researchers are investigating the possibility that neutrinos and dark matter particles may have some underlying connection, potentially shedding light on the nature of both.

In this subchapter, we will explore the latest advancements in neutrino physics and the ongoing experiments designed to unravel the secrets of dark matter. We will discuss the intricate detectors and observatories dedicated to capturing elusive neutrinos and detecting dark matter particles. Furthermore, we will delve into the theoretical frameworks that attempt to explain the properties and behavior of neutrinos and dark matter, providing readers with a comprehensive understanding of these captivating subjects.

Whether you are a curious beginner or an avid particle physics enthusiast, this subchapter will take you on an extraordinary journey through the realm of neutrinos and dark matter. Prepare to be amazed by the wonders of the universe and the frontiers of scientific exploration as we unravel the secrets of these elusive particles.

Chapter 9: Open Questions and Challenges in Neutrino Physics

Neutrino Mass Ordering

In the fascinating world of particle physics, one of the most intriguing mysteries centers around the elusive neutrinos. These subatomic particles are incredibly abundant in the universe, yet they possess some peculiar properties that continue to baffle scientists. One of the most puzzling aspects of neutrinos is their mass and the way it is organized.

Neutrino mass ordering refers to the way in which neutrinos are classified based on their mass values. Just as we have different generations of quarks and charged leptons, neutrinos also come in three flavors: electron neutrinos, muon neutrinos, and tau neutrinos. However, unlike other particles, neutrinos can change their flavor as they travel through space or matter. This phenomenon, known as neutrino oscillation, was a groundbreaking discovery that led to the realization that neutrinos must have mass.

The concept of neutrino mass ordering involves two possibilities: normal ordering and inverted ordering. In normal ordering, the mass of the three neutrinos is arranged in increasing order, with the lightest neutrino being the electron neutrino and the heaviest being the tau neutrino. On the other hand, in inverted ordering, the mass hierarchy is reversed, with the tau neutrino being the lightest and the electron neutrino being the heaviest.

Determining the precise mass ordering of neutrinos is of utmost importance in the field of particle physics. It has significant implications for our understanding of the fundamental laws of nature and the underlying mechanisms at work. The mass ordering of neutrinos provides crucial insights into the nature of neutrino oscillation and the fundamental properties of neutrinos themselves.

Scientists have been conducting numerous experiments to unravel the mystery of neutrino mass ordering. These experiments involve studying neutrino interactions in various contexts, such as underground laboratories and particle accelerators. By carefully analyzing the data obtained from these experiments, researchers aim to decipher the intricate patterns that reveal the true nature of neutrino mass ordering.

Understanding neutrino mass ordering is not only a fundamental pursuit in particle physics but also has broader implications for astrophysics and cosmology. Neutrinos play a vital role in the evolution of the universe, and their masses affect phenomena such as supernovae and the formation of large-scale structures in the cosmos. Therefore, unraveling the mystery of neutrino mass ordering holds the key to unlocking a deeper understanding of the universe itself.

In conclusion, neutrino mass ordering is a captivating and complex topic within the realm of particle physics. Unraveling the arrangement of neutrino masses provides crucial insights into the fundamental nature of these elusive particles and has far-reaching implications for our understanding of the universe. Scientists around the world are dedicated to studying neutrinos and conducting experiments to shed light on this intriguing puzzle, bringing us one step closer to unraveling the mysteries of the subatomic world.

CP Violation in Neutrino Oscillations

Neutrino physics is a fascinating field that delves into the fundamental building blocks of the universe. In this subchapter, we will explore the intriguing phenomenon known as CP violation in neutrino oscillations. This concept plays a crucial role in understanding the behavior of neutrinos and sheds light on the fundamental asymmetry between matter and antimatter in the universe.

Neutrino oscillations occur when neutrinos, which come in three different types or flavors (electron, muon, and tau), morph from one flavor to another as they travel through space. This discovery, made in the late 20th century, revolutionized our understanding of neutrinos and their properties. It also led to the realization that neutrinos have mass, a fact previously unknown to scientists.

CP violation refers to the violation of the combined symmetry of Charge (C) and Parity (P) in the laws of physics. These symmetries state that the fundamental laws of physics should remain the same if we swap particles with their antiparticles (charge symmetry) or if we mirror the entire system (parity symmetry). However, CP violation introduces a subtle imbalance that favors matter over antimatter.

CP violation was first observed in the decays of certain subatomic particles, but its existence in neutrino oscillations presents a unique and exciting opportunity to study this phenomenon further. Neutrinos are elusive particles that interact weakly with matter, making them challenging to study directly. However, experiments conducted over the past few decades have provided strong evidence for CP violation in neutrino oscillations.

The discovery of CP violation in neutrino oscillations has far-reaching implications for particle physics and cosmology. It helps explain why the universe is composed primarily of matter, despite the fact that equal amounts of matter and antimatter should have been produced during the Big Bang. By studying the subtle differences in neutrino oscillations, scientists hope to unravel the mysteries surrounding the asymmetry between matter and antimatter.

Understanding CP violation in neutrino oscillations also has practical applications. It could provide insights into the behavior of neutrinos in astrophysical environments, such as supernovae, where neutrinos play a crucial role. Furthermore, it could have implications for the development of new technologies, such as neutrino detectors and precision measurements, which are essential for advancing our knowledge of fundamental physics.

In conclusion, CP violation in neutrino oscillations is a captivating and significant area of research in particle physics. Its study not only deepens our understanding of neutrinos but also offers insights into the fundamental nature of the universe. By unraveling the mysteries of CP violation, scientists are paving the way for groundbreaking discoveries and advancements in both theoretical and experimental physics.

Neutrino Physics and the Nature of Dark Matter

In the vast realm of particle physics, few subjects are as captivating and mysterious as neutrino physics and the enigmatic nature of dark matter. These two fields, although distinct, share a common thread in their ability to challenge our understanding of the fundamental constituents of the universe. This subchapter aims to shed light on the intricate connections between neutrinos and dark matter, providing a comprehensive overview suitable for both beginners and those seeking advanced knowledge in particle physics.

Neutrinos, often referred to as the "ghost particles" of the universe, are elusive subatomic particles that possess no electric charge and interact weakly with matter. Despite their abundance, neutrinos are notoriously difficult to detect due to their feeble interaction with ordinary matter. Nevertheless, their existence has been firmly established and their study has revolutionized our understanding of particle physics.

Within the realm of neutrino physics lies a fascinating puzzle: the phenomenon of neutrino oscillation. This phenomenon, discovered through meticulous experiments, reveals that neutrinos can change their flavor as they propagate through space. This revelation challenges our previously held notion that neutrinos are massless and uncovers a fundamental gap in our understanding of particle physics. The implications of neutrino oscillation extend beyond their immediate field, influencing theories related to the Higgs boson, the Standard Model, and even the origin of matter in the universe.

Dark matter, on the other hand, presents an entirely different mystery. Unlike neutrinos, which are elusive due to their weak interactions, dark matter is invisible because it does not interact with light or other electromagnetic forces. Its existence is inferred through its gravitational effects on visible matter, yet its nature remains shrouded in uncertainty. What is dark matter made of? Is it composed of exotic particles yet to be discovered? Or does it indicate a breakdown in our understanding of gravity itself?

The subchapter will explore the potential connections between neutrinos and dark matter, investigating the possibility that neutrinos could be involved in the elusive nature of dark matter. Researchers hypothesize that neutrinos, with their weak interactions, could be the key to unraveling the mystery of dark matter, providing valuable insights into its composition and properties.

Whether you are a beginner seeking an introduction to the captivating world of particle physics or an advanced enthusiast looking to delve deeper into the intricate connections between neutrinos and dark matter, this subchapter will serve as an invaluable resource. Prepare to embark on a journey through the subatomic realm, where mysteries are waiting to be unraveled and new frontiers of knowledge are waiting to be explored.

Chapter 10: Conclusion

Summary of Key Concepts

In this subchapter, we will provide a concise summary of the key concepts covered in the book "A Beginner's Guide to Neutrino Physics: From Basics to Advanced Concepts." This summary aims to offer a comprehensive overview of the fundamental principles and advanced concepts in the field of neutrino physics, addressing an audience of both beginners and experts in particle physics.

1. Introduction to Neutrinos: We begin by introducing neutrinos, the elusive subatomic particles that interact weakly with matter. We discuss their properties, such as their charge, mass, and spin, and explain their importance in the study of fundamental particles.

2. Neutrino Oscillations: One of the most remarkable discoveries in neutrino physics is the phenomenon of neutrino oscillations. We delve into the theory behind this phenomenon, which explains how neutrinos change flavor as they travel through space. We explore the experimental evidence supporting this theory and its implications for our understanding of particle physics.

3. Neutrino Interactions: Neutrinos interact very weakly with matter, making their detection and study challenging. We explore the various methods employed to detect neutrinos, including experiments that use large underground detectors and accelerator-based neutrino beams. We also discuss the different types of neutrino interactions, such as elastic scattering and charged-current interactions.

4. Neutrinos in Astrophysics: Neutrinos play a crucial role in astrophysics, providing valuable insights into the inner workings of stars, supernovae, and other cosmic phenomena. We explore the role of neutrinos in stellar nucleosynthesis, their detection from supernovae, and their implications for understanding the early universe.

5. Neutrinos and the Standard Model: The Standard Model of particle physics is the cornerstone of our understanding of fundamental particles and their interactions. We discuss the role of neutrinos within this framework, their connection to other particles, and the challenges they pose to the current understanding of the universe.

6. Neutrino Physics Beyond the Standard Model: The study of neutrinos has also shed light on physics beyond the Standard Model. We explore theories such as sterile neutrinos, neutrino mass hierarchy, and the search for neutrinoless double-beta decay. These advanced concepts push the boundaries of our current understanding and open new avenues for discovery.

By summarizing the key concepts in this subchapter, we hope to provide a solid foundation for readers interested in neutrino physics. Whether you are a beginner seeking an introduction or an expert looking for a comprehensive review, this book aims to satisfy your curiosity and help you navigate the fascinating world of particle physics.

The Future of Neutrino Physics

In this subsection, we provide a comprehensive list of recommended reading materials and references for those interested in delving deeper into the fascinating world of neutrino physics. Whether you are a novice looking to understand the basics or an advanced enthusiast seeking more in-depth knowledge, this collection of resources is tailored to meet your needs.

1. Neutrino Physics: A Beginner's Perspective by J. W. F. Valle and J. C. Romao
As the title suggests, this book offers a beginner-friendly introduction to neutrino physics. It covers the fundamental concepts and experimental techniques, making it an ideal starting point for those new to the field.

2. Neutrino by Frank Close
Written by a renowned physicist, this book provides a comprehensive overview of neutrinos, their properties, and their role in particle physics. It explores the history of neutrino research and discusses the implications of recent discoveries, making it a great choice for both beginners and advanced readers.

3. Neutrino Oscillations: A Practical Guide to Basics and Applications by Igor Gilitsky, Maxim Khlopov, and Sergey Demidov
This text focuses on the phenomenon of neutrino oscillations, a topic of great importance in the field of particle physics. It covers the theoretical aspects of oscillations and their experimental verification.

This book is recommended for readers with a solid foundation in physics and mathematics.

4. Neutrino by Isaak M. Khalatnikov
Providing a historical perspective on the study of neutrinos, this book presents a detailed account of the development of neutrino physics. It covers various aspects of neutrino research, from early discoveries to the latest advancements, making it a valuable resource for readers interested in the historical context of this field.

5. Particle Physics: A Very Short Introduction by Frank Close
This concise yet comprehensive book offers a general overview of particle physics, including the study of neutrinos. It covers the fundamental particles and forces, providing a solid foundation for further exploration in the field. It is recommended for readers with a basic understanding of physics.

6. Review of Particle Physics by Particle Data Group
This widely respected publication compiles the latest experimental results and theoretical developments in particle physics. It offers a comprehensive summary of the field, including neutrino physics. It is an invaluable resource for researchers and advanced students in particle physics.

These recommended reading materials and references cater to readers of all levels of expertise, from beginners seeking a solid introduction to advanced enthusiasts desiring more specialized knowledge. They cover a wide range of topics, including neutrino oscillations, experimental techniques, historical context, and the broader field of particle physics. By exploring these resources, you can gain a deeper understanding of neutrino physics and its significance in the fascinating world of particle physics.

www.ingramcontent.com/pod-product-compliance
Lightning Source LLC
LaVergne TN
LVHW052003060526
838201LV00059B/3815